Ketogenic Diet Plan

30 Day Meal Plan, 50 Ketogenic Fat Burning Recipes for Rapid Weight Loss and Unstoppable Energy

Medical Disclaimer

You understand that any information as found within this book is for general educational and informational purposes only. You understand that such information is not intended nor otherwise implied to be medical advice.

You understand that such information is by no means complete or exhaustive, and that as a result, such information does not encompass all conditions, disorders, health-related issues, or respective treatments. You understand that you should always consult your physician or other healthcare provider to determine the appropriateness of this information for your own situation or should you have any questions regarding a medical condition or treatment plan.

You understand that the products and any related claims for such products have not been evaluated by the United States Food and Drug Administration (USFDA) and are not approved to diagnose, treat, cure or prevent disease. As such, you acknowledge that you are not relying in any fashion that the USFDA has approved of such products and claims.

You agree not to use any information on our book, including, but not limited to product descriptions, customer testimonials, etc. for the diagnosis and treatment of any health issue or for the prescription of any medication or treatment.

You acknowledge that all testimonials as found in our book are strictly the opinion of that person and any results such person may have achieved are solely individual in nature; your results may vary.

You understand that such information is based upon personal experience and is not a substitute for obtaining professional medical advice. You should always consult your physician or other healthcare provider before changing your diet or starting an exercise program.

In light of the forgoing, you understand and agree that we are not liable nor do we assume any liability for any information contained within this book as well as your reliance on it. In no event shall we be liable for direct, indirect, consequential, special, exemplary, or other damages related to your use of the information contained within our book.

This book offers health, fitness and nutritional information and is designed for informational and educational purposes only. You should not rely on this information as a substitute for, nor does it replace, professional medical advice, diagnosis, or treatment. Please discuss all medical and nutrition questions with your health care provider. If you have any concerns or questions about your health, you should always consult with a physician or other health-care professional.

The Food and Drug Administration have not evaluated the statements made within this book. The statements mentioned in this book are not intended to diagnose, treat, cure or prevent any disease.

Do not disregard, avoid or delay obtaining medical or health related advice from your health-care professional because of something you may have read in this book. The use of any information provided in this book is solely at your own risk.

Developments in medical research may impact the health, fitness and nutritional information that appear in this book. No assurance can be given that the information contained in this book will always include the most recent findings or developments with respect to the particular material.

The information provided by this book is believed to be accurate at the time it was created and it was based on research and our best judgment. However, like any printed material, information may become outdated over time. Information on this book may contain technical inaccuracies or typographical errors. Information may be changed or updated without notice.

All users agree that all access to and use of this book is at their own risk. This book or the author does not assume any liability for the information contained herein, be it direct, indirect, consequential, special, exemplary, or other damages; including intangible losses, resulting from: (i) the use or the inability to use our book, our services, or any services or products of any third party; or (ii) statements or conduct of any third party.

If you are in the United States and think you are having a medical or health emergency, call your health care professional, or 911, immediately.

Table of Contents

Introduction

Thank you for taking the time to download this book: Ketogenic Diet Plan: 30 Day Meal Plan, 50 Ketogenic Fat Burning Recipes for Rapid Weight Loss and Unstoppable Energy

This book covers the ketogenic diet plan, and will teach you everything you need to know in order to effectively implement it. It explains the science behind the concept, as well as the side effects and health benefits that come with it. This ketogenic manual also provides a meal plan that you can follow for a month, and a good number of recipes to get you started in preparing keto-friendly meals.

At the completion of this book, you will have a good understanding of what the diet is all about and be able to adapt based on your preferences, weight, and level of physical activity.

Once again, thanks for downloading this book, I hope you find it to be helpful!

Chapter 1 – What is the Ketogenic Diet

The ketogenic diet was originally intended to treat refractory epilepsy in kids, but it's now among the most popular diets around the globe. The diet's mantra is simple – low carbs, enough protein, and high fat. Typically, the body turns the carbohydrates that you get from food into glucose. It is then delivered throughout the body and serves as fuel for your brain and other organs.

With the limited carb intake, the system is forced to burn fat instead. The liver works on the fat and turns it into fatty acids and ketone bodies. The ketone bodies go through the brain and become its energy source in replacement of glucose. When the level of ketone bodies in the blood is raised, the system enters the state of ketosis. This is what sets this kind of diet apart from others, and it's the reason why the diet is effective in reducing the frequency of epileptic seizures.

The diet has five levels – the classic ketogenic diet, modified ketogenic diet, medium-chain triglyceride (MCT) oil supplement diet, low glycemic index treatment (LGIT), and the modified Atkins diet. All these have been proven as effective in treating epilepsy.

The classic ketogenic diet was developed in 1924, by Dr. Russell Wilder, for the treatment of pediatric epilepsy and was widely used in the following years. In the 1940s, the popularity of the diet suffered as new anti-seizure medications were introduced. It was revived in 1994 when Jim Abrahams, a Hollywood producer, started the Charlie

Foundation. It was testament to how the diet worked for Jim's child, Charlie. The latter started to undergo the ketogenic diet when he was a toddler and kept the lifestyle for the next five years. It came after several failed attempts in trying other anti-seizure medications and undergoing brain surgery. Charlie served as proof of how effective this diet can be in controlling severe epilepsy.

It was the foundation's goal to bring awareness about this diet to more people. It was done through publicity materials and by sponsoring a multicenter prospective study. The study announced its results in 1996, which paved the way for the renewed interest about the diet.

The Basics

If you choose to follow the ketogenic diet, you will have to reduce your daily intake of carbs to 20-60 grams. The amount of protein that you have to consume, on the other hand, will depend on your gender, height, and the physical activities you do every day. You need to balance the amount of calories in your daily diet based on your protein and carb requirements.

However, his kind of diet does not necessarily require you to count the calories from everything you eat. It is more important to be aware of the percentages of the macronutrients that you are getting. They can greatly be affected by very high or low calorie intake. Your daily intake ratio (in terms of caloric distribution) has to be composed of around 25 percent protein, up to 10 percent carbs, and 70-75 percent fat.

How does a moderate protein and high-fat kind of diet work? Fats have a very limited effect on your insulin and blood sugar levels, but both of these are highly affected by your protein intake. When you consume too much protein, the tendency is for your blood sugar and insulin levels to rise temporarily. This will slow down the body's production of ketones. When you continue to eat more protein without getting enough fat, you may end up suffering from rabbit starvation and this can also slow down your metabolism. Rabbit starvation was a term coined by American explorers when they had very little access to carbohydrates and fats and ate only very lean meat such as rabbits and small game.

Is the Diet Dangerous?

The popularity of the ketogenic diet brought a lot of fallacies and myths. Make sure that you don't fall into the following fears. Understand the process and its benefits before you make your own conclusions.

A lot of people doubt the benefits of taking in a high amount of fat because they grew up thinking that it's bad for your health. Fat doesn't make you fat, but sugar does. You'll get a high dose of sugar when you maintain a high-carb kind of diet. Saturated fat could be healthy, but when combined with high sugar, you will suffer from inflammation that may lead to heart ailments. The aim of the ketogenic diet is to reduce that inflammation through reduced carbohydrate consumption and increased saturated fat intake.

In the ketogenic diet, the high amount of saturated fat that you take boosts the level of the good cholesterol or HDL and decreases you triglycerides levels. This makes your heart healthier and it reduces your risks of suffering from related diseases.

Before you begin with the diet, it is recommended to get a full blood test. You must also ask for your doctor's approval, especially if you are under any kind of medication or therapy. If you are qualified to proceed, follow the diet for three months and have your blood checked again. This duration is enough for you to know how your body has benefited from the process.

Why is it important to get your blood checked? Not everybody has the same reaction to ketosis, especially those who are prone or already suffering from heart disease and kidney problems. To be safe even if you have the best of health, never go lower than 10 grams of carbs per day. This is not a zero-carb kind of diet. Your body will actually tell you if it needs more carbs. Listen to it and abide by its needs by gradually adding to your carb intake without going overboard.

The Side Effects

This diet, like any kind of diet plan, has temporary side effects. They will naturally go away after your body has adjusted to what you are eating. Do not get disheartened by them. Always bear in mind that the number of benefits of the ketogenic diet outweighs its side effects, which include the following:

1. Frequent urination. This happens in the first week as the system burns the stored glucose or the extra glycogen in the muscles and liver. The process releases a lot of water and your kidneys will dump the excess liquid. The kidneys also begin to excrete excess sodium since you won't have as much insulin being circulated in your bloodstream.

2. Dizziness. When you urinate frequently, your system loses not only too much liquid, but also minerals, such as magnesium, salt and potassium. This leads to feeling lightheaded and dizzy. It's also likely that you'll get tired easily. For some people, this may result to headaches, itchiness of the skin, and muscle cramps.

This kind of side effect can be avoided. You already know what can lead to this, so you can counteract the mineral loss beforehand. This can be done by adding more salt into your diet and eating foods rich in potassium, such as avocados, dairy, and green leafy vegetables.

When you get below 60 grams of carbs each day, make sure that you take in a moderate amount of salt (up to 5 grams a day). It is also ideal to take 400 mg of magnesium citrate at night before you sleep. If you are suffering from high blood pressure and other heart ailments, consult with your doctor before implementing the changes. To get a good dose of vitamin K and potassium, eat at least two cups of raw green leafy veggies each day. Aside from supplementing the nutrients that your body needs, they will also help in suppressing your appetite.

3. Low Blood Sugar or Hypoglycemia. This is your body's initial reaction to the sudden drop in carbohydrate intake.

4. Sugar cravings. The cravings will range from bad to worse for two up to 21 days. This duration is considered as the transition period. No matter how hard it is to resist carbs, make sure that you don't cheat. Cheating will stop your progress and will make it harder to avoid carbs in the future. There are a lot of recipes, which are going to be discussed in the latter part of this book, that you can try to make yourself feel that you are not missing out on anything. You simply need to be creative in the pairings of your dishes and in how you prepare your food.

5. Headaches. You'll likely experience this for several days. The roots of the problem is the loss of minerals

in your diet. If you want to test if the headache is due to sodium loss, add ¼ teaspoon of salt in a glass of water, mix and drink it. This will relieve you of the headache in less than 30 minutes. As you go through your diet, drink more fluids and take in more salt, if your health permits.

6. Constipation. When you suffer from this, you will also likely get tired and dizzy. If it happens too often and the magnesium citrate is not helping, you can cut back your consumption of dairy products. You can also cut back on the amount of nuts that you are eating and make sure that you take in lots of fluids.

7. Diarrhea. This is common in any diet plan. It happens as the body tries to adjust to what you are feeding it with. This will naturally go away in a matter of days. It might help to take a teaspoon of plain psyllium husk powder or sugar-free Metamucil before a meal. They contain fiber that will absorb excess fluid in your colon and work on your loose stools.

8. Feeling weak and shaky. This happens due to lower levels of sugar that your body is getting. You can counteract the effect by adding a little more protein and salt in your diet. You can also take potassium citrate supplements, but never take more than what's recommended. You have to get most of your potassium requirements from the food that you eat. Remember that having too much potassium isn't good for the heart.

9. Muscle cramps. This side effect is again due to the loss of minerals. You can take three slow-release magnesium tablets each day at the beginning and if the side effect continues after 20 days, limit the intake to one tablet each day.

10. Difficulty sleeping. It may be hard for you to stay asleep due to the low levels of insulin and serotonin in your system. To counter this side effect, snack on something that contains protein and a little carb before you hit the bed. The carb will increase your insulin that will prompt more tryptophan that you can get from protein, to get absorbed by your brain. Tryptophan has a soothing effect that will ease out your sleeping troubles. A good combination of snack that you can try is Greek yogurt with a little square of 70% chocolate or half a tablespoon of fruit spread.

11. Heart palpitations. This may happen for a week or up to two months after you have started with the diet. People with low blood pressure are more prone to this. To prevent you from experiencing this, it is recommended to take a multivitamin that contains the RDA for magnesium, zinc, and selenium. Make sure that you drink lots of fluids, specifically mineral water.

    This side effect may also be due to medium MCT oil or excessive coconut oil consumption. You have to gradually add these oils in your diet. You must also add other oils in your diet, such as ghee, animal fats, butter and olive oil.

    This can also be due to your activity levels. In this case, your system may need more protein. Gradually add 5 to 10 grams of protein in your every meal.

12. Hair Loss. This is another side effect that is common in almost all kinds of diet. It happens due to the changes in hormone levels and metabolism. This kind of hair loss is referred to as telogen effluvium. It's only temporary and will eventually subside once your body has adapted to the diet.

Chapter 2 – Your Body During Ketosis

What's so special about ketosis and why is it considered as the major advantage of this diet? Ketosis is a metabolic state in which your system relies on the ketone bodies in the blood for energy. This is a normal process that your body enters when it lacks carbohydrates and it has a high fat-burning rate.

Women who begin exercising after pregnancy also typically experience this. This carries a different meaning when you have uncontrolled diabetes. In this case, it signals that your system is already lacking its required amount of insulin. This is the reason why this kind of diet is not recommended for those who have type-1 diabetes that is insulin dependent.

The production of ketones is encouraged by reducing the amount of insulin in your bloodstream. The higher your ketone production is, the lower your insulin levels will be – but you'll have greater chances of achieving optimal ketosis. The build-up of ketones can also become dangerous. This is the reason why the food and nutrients in the diet are controlled. Extremely high levels of ketones may cause a chemical imbalance in the blood, which may lead to dehydration.

This metabolic state is an effective strategy to lose weight. As it burns your body fats, you will feel less hungry and it will be easier to develop and maintain muscles. For as long as you are healthy (and that you aren't pregnant and you don't have diabetes), your body will begin entering this state within three to four days after you have started with the low-carb diet. Your body will also enter this state through fasting.

How does it help those who are suffering from epilepsy?

Children respond to ketosis by having less or no seizures at all after undergoing a special high-fat and low protein and carb diet scheme. For adults who have the disorder, they are advised to follow the modified Atkins diet to improve their health. Through continued research, it was found out that the diet also helps in improving a lot of health conditions, which include heart ailments, cancer, Parkinson's disease, Lou Gehrig's disease, Alzheimer's, and a lot more.

How do you test your ketones?

There are test strips that you can buy to check your urine at home in order to test your ketones. You can also use certain blood sugar meters to check your blood. There is no need to go to the doctor, unless you are unsure about the process or your body is not responding well to the diet.

- Blood ketones ought to be measured in the morning before you eat anything. If the result is below 0.5 mmol/L, you still haven't achieved ketosis and you're actually far from getting the maximum effects of fat-burning. You have attained a light nutritional ketosis if the result is between 0.5-1.5 mmol/L, but this will not yield optimal results if you aim to lose weight. You will gain optimal ketosis if the result is at around 1.5-3 mmol/L. Higher values could mean danger if you are a diabetic, but if not, they may indicate that you are not eating enough.

- The ketone sticks that are used to test the urine are not as reliable as the blood tests, but they are cheaper and easier to follow.

When you get high levels of ketosis, the ketones in your blood build up and become acidic. This is referred to as ketoacidosis, which is dangerous and can cause comatose or death. Those who have type-1 diabetes are more prone to this when they don't get enough insulin, they become sick or get dehydrated due to lack of fluid intake. Those who don't have diabetes can also suffer from this due to starvation, overactive thyroid, and alcoholism.

Here are some signs that you may already be nearing a ketone build-up. Do not wait until it is too late before you call a doctor:

- Feeling dazed and confused
- Frequent urination
- Having difficulty breathing
- Dry skin
- Dry mouth and the feeling that you are always thirsty
- Stomach ache
- Throwing up
- Your breath has a weird fruity smell

Throwing up can be especially harmful to those who have diabetes because it can speed up the process of having ketoacidosis in only a few hours. Seek help from your doctor if you don't stop throwing up within two hours.

How to Achieve Optimal Ketosis

Your goal is to achieve optimal ketosis in order to lose weight. You have to be careful with what you eat. Aside from avoiding foods that are rich in carbs, such as bread, pastas, sweets, potatoes and rice, you must also be careful when it comes to your protein intake. Make sure that you don't get too much protein, or else, your insulin levels will get higher as the excess protein is turned into glucose.

Whenever you eat, fill your cravings with fat. For example, douse your steak with a big helping of herb butter. This will make you feel so full that you won't reach for another serving. Many people who are undergoing the diet do the trick with how they prepare coffee. In order to ingest more fat, you can add a tablespoon of butter and a tablespoon of coconut oil to your morning coffee. You will eventually get used to the taste, but to make the consistency more fluid, you can process this in a food blender. When you get more fat into your system, the tendency is to eat less protein and even lesser carbs. This will result to the drop of your insulin levels and will make it easier for you to experience optimal ketosis.

Chapter 3 – What Are the Health Benefits of a Ketogenic Diet

It's important that you don't simply lose weight when you're on a diet. After all, your ultimate goal should be to live a healthier life and attain overall wellbeing. To prove that the ketogenic diet isn't a mere weight-loss solution, here are some of its most vital health benefits:

1. It will suppress your appetite. Many people give up on their diets because they can no longer contain their hunger. Ketogenic diet allows you to experience an automatic reduction of your food cravings. Even though you won't feel hungry, this doesn't mean that you will stop eating. You have to eat according to the plan and make sure that you take the kinds of foods that are appropriate for this diet.

When you eat more protein and fat than carbs, the tendency is to take in fewer calories. This is hard to do with certain kinds of diets and will require rigorous calorie counting in every food that you eat or ingredient that you buy. With this diet, you will end up taking in less calories without even trying. It goes hand in hand with the kinds of food that this diet requires.

2. This will allow you to lose weight in a safe and effective manner. The diet helps in getting rid of the excess water in your system. Your kidneys will begin to shed excess sodium as you achieve lower levels of insulin. This will result in rapid weight loss within one to two weeks.

You will continue to lose weight for up to six months. At this point, your goal will be to maintain the kind of figure that you have already achieved. This is easier said than done and many people have already failed because after this period, they tend to go back to eating the food that they used to eat before they followed the diet. Once you gave in to the temptation, it will be hard to go back to dieting. You have to remember that maintenance is harder than the process of losing weight. You must always have the discipline to eat in moderation and avoid food that will boost your weight. Make the diet part of your lifestyle and not as a mere solution to lose weight for a limited period of time.

3. The diet reduces harmful abdominal fat. Not all kinds of fats in your body carry the same dangers and risks. It all depends on where these fats are stored. The body has subcutaneous fat, which is located under the skin and visceral fat, which is stored in the abdominal cavity. The latter lodges onto your organs, which can lead to inflammation.

The ketogenic diet works by getting rid of abdominal fat. Aside from allowing you to get fit, this will also help in reducing your chances of developing type-2 diabetes. If you will allow your abdominal fat to get bigger and you don't do anything about it, you will likely experience severe metabolic problems that can lead to other health disorders.

4. Your triglyceride levels will go down. They are fat molecules and the higher levels of these that you have in the blood, the greater your chances of having heart ailments. The levels of these fat molecules elevate with the consumption of carbs and simple sugar fructose. You will experience a drastic reduction in triglyceride levels when you begin cutting carbs from your diet.

5. You will have increased levels of good cholesterol or HDL.

6. This will lead to the reduced levels of insulin and blood sugar in your system. The carbs that you eat are broken down by the digestive tract into simple sugars and glucose. They will go through your bloodstream and may elevate your blood sugar levels. Since this state can be toxic, the body responds by releasing insulin and forcing glucose to get either stored or burned. This is okay for healthy individuals, but there are certain people who are insulin resistant. If you are among them, your cells will not recognize the insulin and your system will find it difficult to bring the blood sugar into the cells.

If it continues and you don't do anything to prevent it, this can develop into type-2 diabetes. This condition is common these days and is said to affect around 300 million people around the world. The solution is easy and the ketogenic diet has laid it all out – cut the carbs and eat more fat. The diet will not make your system dependent on glucose. You will be able to remove the need for higher levels of insulin. As you go on with the diet, both your insulin and blood sugar levels will go down.

The diet is actually being applied these days by many doctors in treating diabetic patients. This enables them to drastically reduce the insulin dosage of their patients to 50 percent. There are studies which prove that more than 95 percent of people with type-2 diabetes are able to eliminate or reduce their glucose-lowering medications six months after they have started with the diet.

Chapter 4 – Foods to Eat in Ketosis

Going on a diet is never easy. To make the process a little less complicated, you ought to know beforehand the right foods to eat. This way, you will know what to shop for whenever you hit the grocery store.

Here are the right foods that can help you achieve the state of ketosis:

1. Protein

The protein sources in your diet must be organic and grass-fed, if available. The products from these sources will lessen your chances of taking in steroid hormone and bacteria.

- Whole eggs. It is better if you can get them free-range from your local market. You will never run out of ways to prepare your eggs. You can have them boiled or fried. You can also get more creative and serve them with salads and desserts.
- Shellfish. The best protein sources of this type include lobster, squid, scallops, clams, mussels, crabs and oysters.
- Fish. You can eat just about anything that is caught wild. Some samples of good varieties of fish include salmon, tuna, catfish, mackerel, snapper, flounder, cod, halibut, trout, and mahi-mahi.
- Meat. As much as possible, choose the grass-fed kind because this contains more fatty acids. You can have meat from lamb, veal, goat, and beef. For pork, you can choose pork chops and pork loins. You can also eat ham, but avoid the kinds with added sugars.

- Poultry. Choose organic and free range types of poultry meat, such as chicken, quail, pheasant, and duck
- Peanut butter. Choose the natural type, but make sure that you take this in moderation because it contains high doses of carbs and Omega-6. It is healthier and safer to choose macadamia nut butter.
- Sausage and bacon. Make sure that you only get the type with no fillers and added sugars.

2. Fats and Oils

Your body needs a high dose of fats to aid in digestion. You will also be getting your daily calorie intake from these sources. They are important in achieving ketosis, but always make sure that you are getting the right kinds. Consuming the wrong types of fats can take a toll on your health. It is your goal to maintain a balance between Omega-3 and Omega-6. Omega-3 can be found in seafood, such as shellfish, tuna, trout and salmon. If you don't like fish, you can get your Omega-3 by taking a fish oil supplement.

Many people will benefit from saturated and monounsaturated fats that are less inflammatory and more chemically stable. Some examples include macadamia nuts, egg yolks, avocado, coconut oil, and butter. These fats and oils can be served in a variety of ways. They can be added to your meals and beverages, or used as dressings or sauces.

As much as possible, avoid hydrogenated fats in order to minimize the trans-fat that you get into your system. A good example of this is margarine. Consuming a lot of hydrogenated fats make you more at risk of developing coronary heart disease. When using vegetable oils, such as safflower, soybean, flax and olive, look for the cold pressed variety as much as possible.

To get more essential fatty acids from fried food, use non-hydrogenated lard, which has a higher smoke points as compared to other oils. Omega-6 can be found mostly on seeds and nuts, such as pine nuts, walnuts and almonds, and oils that include corn and sunflower. Make sure that you take them in moderation because too much of these can cause inflammation.

When shopping for fats and oils, prioritize the organic types and products that come from grass-fed sources. Here are some of the best sources of fats and oils that can help you in achieving ketosis:

- Non-hydrogenated lard
- Avocado
- Coconut butter
- Chicken fat
- Macadamia nuts
- Beef tallow
- Mayonnaise
- Olive oil
- Ghee
- Peanut butter
- Butter
- Coconut oil
- Red palm oil

3. Dairy products

Choose the kinds that are full-fat and find the types that are organic and raw, as much as you can. Here's a look at how much calories, fats, net carbs, and protein (in that particular order) you get for every ounce of the following dairy products:

- Buttermilk – 18, 0.9 gram, 1.4 grams, and 0.9 gram
- Feta cheese – 75, 6 grams, 1.2 grams, and 4 grams
- Monterey Jack cheese – 106, 8.6 grams, 0.2 gram, and 7 grams
- Cottage cheese (2%) – 24, 0.7 gram, 1 gram, and 3.3 grams
- Blue cheese – 100, 8.2 grams, 0.7 gram, and 6.1 grams
- Colby cheese – 110, 9 grams, 0.7 gram, and 6.7 grams
- Cheddar cheese – 114, 9.4 grams, 0.4 gram and 7.1 grams
- Brie cheese – 95, 7.9 grams, 0.1 gram, and 5.9 grams
- Mozzarella cheese – 85, 6.3 grams, 0.6 gram, and 6.3 grams
- Parmesan cheese (hard) – 111, 7.3 grams, 0.9 gram, and 10.1 grams
- Swiss cheese – 108, 7.9 grams, 1.5 grams, and 7.6 grams
- Cream cheese (block) – 97, 9.7 grams, 1.1 grams, and 1.7 grams
- Mascarpone cheese – 130, 13 grams, 1 gram, and 1 gram
- Heavy cream – 103, 11 grams, 0.8 gram, and 0.6 gram
- Half-n-half cream – 39, 3.5 grams, 1.3 grams, and 0.9 gram
- Sour cream (full fat) – 55, 5.6 grams, 0.8 gram, and 0.6 gram
- Whole milk – 19, 1 gram, 1.5 grams, and 1 gram
- Skim milk – 10, 0, 1.5 grams, and 1 gram
- Milk (2%) – 15, 0.6 gram, 1.5 grams, and 1 gram

4. Vegetables

The best veggies are those grown above the ground, particularly leafy greens. It would better if you can get the organic types since they don't contain pesticide residue. It is okay if you can't have find organic veggies, the non-organic kinds still contain the same nutritional qualities. You simply need to clean them thoroughly before preparing and cooking.

Not all kinds of vegetables are suited for the ketogenic diet. Make sure that you stay away from the kinds that are high in sugar. You have to fill your plate with those that are low in carbs and have high nutritional content. Avoid vegetables that are starchy and have a high content of carbohydrates, such as potatoes, yams, beans, legumes, yucca, corn, parsnips and peas. You simply have to think that the sweet vegetable varieties contain more sugar, so you need to avoid them as much as you can. You can still eat them in moderation, especially since most of these veggies make dishes more flavorful. These veggies include peppers, squash, onion and carrot.

Here's a list of vegetables that are suited for this diet and how much net carbs you get for every serving of 1/2 cup:

- Mustard greens – 0.1
- Raw spinach – 0.1
- Chopped parsley – 0.1
- Romaine lettuce – 0.2
- Iceberg lettuce – 0.2
- Bok Choi – 0.2
- Endive – 0.2
- Sprouts Alfalfa – 0.2
- Boston Bibb lettuce – 0.4
- Boiled turnips greens – 0.6

- Radicchio – 0.7
- Broccoli florets – 0.8
- Steamed cauliflower 0.9
- Jalapeño pepper – 1
- Grilled nopales – 1
- Raw cucumber – 1
- Cooked zucchini – 1
- Cooked shitake mushroom – 1.1
- Raw green cabbage – 1.1
- Summer squash – 1.3
- Raw red cabbage – 1.4
- Button mushroom – 1.4
- Raw cauliflower – 1.4
- Steamed zucchini squash – 1.5
- Steamed green cabbage – 1.6
- Fresh fennel – 1.8
- Steamed savoy cabbage – 1.9
- Collard greens – 2
- Broccoli rabe – 2
- Sauerkraut – 2.1
- Broiled eggplant – 2.1
- Bean sprouts – 2.1
- Steamed kale – 2.1
- Steamed spinach – 2.2
- Boiled turnips – 2.3
- Raw jicama – 2.4
- Scallions – 2.4

5. Seeds and nuts

To get rid of the anti-nutrients of these foods, it is best to have them roasted. Avoid peanuts as much as you can. They are not really considered nuts, but legumes and are not preferred in this kind of diet plan.

Here's a look at how much calories, fat, net carbs, and protein (in that particular order) you get for every ounce serving of the following raw nuts and seeds:

- Cashews – 160, 13 grams, 7 grams, and 5 grams
- Chia seeds – 131, 10 grams, 0 grams, and 7 grams
- Almonds – 170, 15 grams, 3 grams, and 6 grams
- Chestnuts – 55, 0 grams, 13 grams, and 0 grams
- Flax seeds – 131, 10 grams, 0 grams, and 7 grams
- Coconut (dried and unsweetened) – 65, 6 grams, 2 grams, and 1 gram
- Hazelnuts – 176, 17 grams, 2 grams, and 4 grams
- Macadamia nuts – 203, 21 grams, 2 grams, and 2 grams
- Pine nuts – 189, 20 grams, 3 grams, and 4 grams
- Brazil nuts – 186, 19 grams, 1 gram, and 4 grams
- Pistachios – 158, 13 grams, 5 grams, and 6 grams
- Pumpkin seeds – 159, 14 grams, 1 gram, and 8 grams
- Pecans – 190, 20 grams, 1 gram, and 3 grams
- Sunflower seeds – 150, 11 grams, 4 grams, and 3 grams
- Sesame seeds – 160, 14 grams, 4 grams, and 5 grams
- Walnuts – 185, 18 grams, 2 grams, and 4 grams

Again, nuts contain high amounts of Omega-6 fatty acids, so take them in moderation. Cashews and pistachios are specifically higher in carb content as compared to the other nuts. Your best choices of nuts include walnuts, almonds and macadamias, but you must still eat them in small amounts. Instead of using regular flour for baking, you can use nut and seed flours, such as milled flax seed and almond flour.

6. Beverages

This diet has a natural diuretic effect. You have to drink lots of fluids to avoid dehydration, especially in the beginning. Aside from taking in plenty of water, you can also drink herbal and non-herbal teas, and coffee.

7. Sweeteners

If you have to use artificial sweeteners, it is better to choose those in liquid form. They don't contain added binders, which can add to your carb intake. Your best options include the liquid forms of stevia and sucralose, and other sweeteners, such as xylitol, agave nectar, erythritol, and monk fruit.

8. Spices

Be careful in using spices because they contain carbs and many pre-made types have added sugars. To spice up your dishes, you can use the following in moderation: sea salt, basil, black pepper, cumin, cinnamon, parsley, cayenne pepper, thyme, oregano, cilantro, chili powder, turmeric, sage, and rosemary.

Chapter 5 – Physical Performance on the Ketogenic Diet

With the low carb intake that this diet requires, some people fear, especially those who are involved in a lot of physical activities, that it might affect their performance. This has led to studies done by various groups and individuals from the different parts of the world.

One of the most recent studies was done in Italy. It aims to find out how the diet influences explosive strength performance. It analyzed the body composition and different aspects of physical performance of eight elite artistic gymnasts after going through the modified ketogenic diet for a month.

These gymnasts were made to perform the following movements for the study: pushups, pullups, hanging leg raise, squat jumps, parallel bar dips, countermovement jumps, and continuous jumps for 30 seconds. They went on with their usual training and were tested again after 3 months.

With the modified diet, the meals was composed of cooked and raw vegetables, eggs, cheese, poultry, veal, fish and beef, and cold cuts, such as cured ham, dried beef and carpaccio. Aside from water, they were allowed to drink mocha coffee, infusion tea, and herbal extracts. They were not allowed to have pasta, yogurt, bread, rice, milk, barley coffee, alcohol, and soluble tea.

After the trial period, they were placed under a different kind of diet and were allowed to eat the usual foods that they used to take. Their meals include whole grains, such as rice, whole wheat, bread and pasta, eggs, meat and poultry, potatoes, fruits, whole milk, wine, vegetables, legumes, and olive oil. Their physical performance was again.tested before and after 30 days.

Here are the valuable findings from the study:

- There were no substantial differences in the basal physical performance before and after the athletes have gone through both kinds of diet plans.
- The major changes that were seen when they have undergone the modified ketogenic diet include the reduction of the fat percentage, fat mass, and body weight, as well as a significant increase in lean body mass percentage. No significant changes were noted after they have gone through the second type of diet plan.

The study showed that despite the significant weight loss, you can still maintain your body's strength and power when you undergo a modified ketogenic diet. You may feel weak in the beginning, but you will get the hang of it as you progress with the diet and as your body becomes more keto-adapted.

Chapter 6 – 30-Day Ketogenic Meal Plan

When you are ready to undergo the ketogenic diet, you must bear in mind that the beginning is the hardest part. Exert more effort in avoiding temptations and in sticking to the plan.

Week 1

Make everything simple and be creative in tweaking your leftovers. You must also be prepared to suffer from the common side effects and learn to counter most of these as much as you can.

It is ideal to begin the diet on a weekend. This way, you will have ample time to prepare most of the meals that you will consume for the week. For breakfast, you will want meals that are tasty and easy to prepare, including the leftovers. Lunch will be mostly composed of meats and salads with high-fat dressings. There will be limited meat for dinner, but lots of leafy greens. For the first two weeks, stay away from having snacks or desserts.

Day 1 – the following meals will yield a total of 142.5 grams of fats, 72.6 grams of protein, 1596 calories, and 6.5 grams net carbs.

- Breakfast – Scrambled eggs with cheese
- Lunch – Spinach salad and inside out bacon burger
- Dinner – Orange and cinnamon beef stew

Day 2 – the following meals will yield a total of 139.8 grams of fats, 77.8 grams of protein, 1601 calories, and 7.7 grams net carbs.

- Breakfast - 2 Frittata muffins
- Lunch – Spinach salad and canned chicken
- Dinner – Leftover inside out bacon burger and red pepper salad

Day 3 – the following meals will yield a total of 136 grams of fats, 75.5 grams of protein, 1602 calories, and 12.8 grams net carbs.

- Breakfast – 2 Frittata muffins
- Lunch – Spinach salad and chicken sausage
- Dinner – Cauliflower and shrimp curry

Day 4 – the following meals will yield a total of 134 grams of fats, 72.6 grams of protein, 1604 calories, and 4.1 grams net carbs.

- Breakfast – 2 Frittata muffins
- Lunch – Spinach salad and no meat
- Dinner – 1 Curry-rubbed chicken thigh and fried Queso Fresco

Day 5 – the following meals will yield a total of 140g grams of fats, 76.7 grams of protein, 1580 calories, and 10.5 grams net carbs.

- Breakfast – Scrambled eggs with cheese
- Lunch – Spinach salad and leftover curry-rubbed chicken thigh
- Dinner – Stir-fried bacon and sausage, and chicken

Day 6 – the following meals will yield a total of 136.1 grams of fats, 77.1 grams of protein, 1594 calories, and 12.8 grams net carbs.

- Breakfast – Scrambled eggs with cheese with extra butter
- Lunch – Spinach salad with cream cheese

- Dinner – Bacon-infused sugar snap peas and 1/4 serving of Not Your Caveman Chili dish

Day 7 – the following meals will yield a total of 137 grams of fats, 74.7 grams of protein, 1602 calories, and 8.8 grams net carbs.

- Breakfast – Scrambled eggs with cheese
- Lunch – Spinach salad and canned chicken
- Dinner – Cheddar and chorizo meatballs and roasted pecan green beans

Week 2

The breakfast remains simple, but for this week, you have to get yourself used to the taste of a bulletproof coffee. It means that you have to mix butter, heavy cream, and coconut oil into your regular coffee. If you can't take the taste, you can try adding the same ingredients to your tea. If you still can't take it, you can eat the added ingredients while drinking your coffee. This coffee will boost your energy for the rest of the day. You can also add sweeteners, if you prefer. For this week, lunch and dinner are composed of meat, leftovers, and green veggies with vinaigrettes and high-fat dressings. There are still no snacks or desserts for this week.

Day 8 – the following meals will yield a total of 135.8 grams of fats, 79.9 grams of protein, 1605 calories, and 10.2 grams net carbs.

- Breakfast – Bulletproof coffee
- Lunch – Spinach salad and omnivore burger
- Dinner – Bacon and mozzarella meatballs and roasted pecan green beans

Day 9 – the following meals will yield a total of 136.5 grams of fats, 66.5 grams of protein, 1577 calories, and 11.8 grams net carbs.

- Breakfast – Bulletproof coffee
- Lunch – Spinach salad and 1 chicken thigh
- Dinner – Bacon-infused sugar snap peas and buffalo chicken strips

Day 10 – the following meals will yield a total of 135 grams of fats, 78.8 grams of protein, 1607 calories, and 17.2 grams net carbs.

- Breakfast – Bulletproof coffee
- Lunch – Chive, bacon and cheddar mug cake
- Dinner – 2 servings of shrimp and cauliflower curry with extra butter

Day 11 – the following meals will yield a total of 134.2 grams of fats, 74.5 grams of protein, 1610 calories, and 9.9 grams net carbs.

- Breakfast – Bulletproof coffee
- Lunch – Spinach salad and canned chicken
- Dinner – Roasted pecan green beans and 6 Chorizo meatballs

Day 12 – the following meals will yield a total of 133.5 grams of fats, 76.4 grams of protein, 1577 calories, and 11.2 grams net carbs.

- Breakfast – Bulletproof coffee
- Lunch – 2 Keto-friendly taco tartlets
- Dinner – 2 curry-rubbed chicken thighs and red pepper spinach salad

Day 13 – the following meals will yield a total of 140.8 grams of fats, 83.9 grams of protein, 1671 calories, and 10.6 grams net carbs.

- Breakfast – Bulletproof coffee
- Lunch – Chicken strip sliders
- Dinner – Almond flax slider bun and omnivore burger with creamed spinach

Day 14 – the following meals will yield a total of 130.5 grams of fats, 77.9 grams of protein, 1555 calories, and 12.4 grams net carbs.

- Breakfast – Bulletproof coffee
- Lunch – Spinach salad and Mozzarella meatballs
- Dinner – Stir fried bacon and sausage, and chicken

Week 3

The good news for this week is that there are going to be some desserts, but the catch is, there will be no lunch. You need to undergo a slight fast for this week. You will get a fill of fats in the morning and fast till dinner time. To make it easier for you to adjust, have your breakfast at 7AM and set your dinner at 7PM. There should be at least 12 hours in between the two meals in order to keep your body in a fasted state. In this state, your system is able to break down the extra fat to provide energy for your body. If you find this hard and you cannot last a day without having all the major meals, you can skip the list and go back to the week 1 meal plan.

Since you won't be eating lunch, stay hydrated by drinking plenty of water. This will also keep you up until the next meal.

Day 15 – the following meals will yield a total of 150.7 grams of fats, 65 grams of protein, 1577 calories, and 10.7 grams net carbs.

- Breakfast – Double serving of bulletproof coffee
- Dinner – A portion of cheddar bacon explosion, 4 cups of spinach, and a slice of low-carb spice cake for dessert

Day 16 – the following meals will yield a total of 156 grams of fats, 65.3 grams of protein, 1694 calories, and 7.1 grams net carbs.

- Breakfast – Double serving of bulletproof coffee
- Dinner – Inside out bacon burger with 3 patties and a slice of low-carb spice cake for dessert

Day 17 – the following meals will yield a total of 150.7 grams of fats, 62 grams of protein, 1549 calories, and 9.7 grams net carbs.

- Breakfast – Double serving of bulletproof coffee
- Dinner – A portion of cheddar bacon explosion and a slice of low-carb spice cake for dessert

Day 18 – the following meals will yield a total of 135 grams of fats, 80.7 grams of protein, 1578 calories, and 12.8 grams net carbs.

- Breakfast – Double serving of bulletproof coffee
- Dinner – 1 1/3 serving of Not Your Caveman Chili dish and 3 vanilla latte cookies for dessert

Day 19 – the following meals will yield a total of 132.9 grams of fats, 79.4 grams of protein, 1599 calories, and 6.4 grams net carbs.

- Breakfast – Double serving of bulletproof coffee

- Dinner – Chicken pesto roulade, 1/4 pound fried Queso Fresco, 4 cups of spinach, and 1 vanilla latte cookie for dessert

Day 20 – the following meals will yield a total of 144.2 grams of fats, 70.3 grams of protein, 1636 calories, and 10.6 grams net carbs.

- Breakfast – Double serving of bulletproof coffee
- Dinner – Red spinach salad, 1/4 portion of the Simple keto BBQ pulled chicken recipe, and 2 vanilla latte cookies for dessert

Day 21 – the following meals will yield a total of 144.3 grams of fats, 82.5 grams of protein, 1670 calories, and 5 grams net carbs.

- Breakfast – Double serving of bulletproof coffee
- Dinner – 1/3 pound of fried Queso, 80 percent of the Bacon wrapped pork tenderloin recipe and a slice of low-carb spice cake for dessert

Week 4

You've undergone intermittent fasting the past week. For this week, it's going to be stricter, but hold on because you're almost there. After this week, you can plan for complete meals, coupled with snacks and desserts. Just make sure that you remain faithful to the right foods and eat everything in moderation.

Whenever you crave for food and it is nowhere near dinner time, drink lots of fluids. Bring water anywhere you go. Aside from water, you can also drink tea, coffee and flavored water. It is important to remember that you cannot have more than 3 cups of tea or coffee for each day. At the beginning of this week, expect a lot of growling from your stomach. Fill it with fluids and through the days, the noises will stop as your body learns to adjust to the diet.

If you did not fast on the third week, skip this meal plan and follow the one for week two. Not everybody can fast. Only those who have sheer control and determination can last through it, though managing to succeed brings many health benefits.

Fasting begins as soon as you wake up. You can set a time when you will begin and stop eating. For example, you can do it from 5 or 6 in the afternoon, until 11 at night. This will make you feel full until the next day. This will make you look forward to dinner. First, break your fast with a small snack. You can then have a meal after 30 minutes or so and have another until you are satisfied. Here's the plan for the week:

Day 22 – the following meals will yield a total of 119.6 grams of fats, 80.2 grams of protein, 1558 calories, and 20 grams net carbs.

- Breakfast and lunch – Plenty of water. You can also drink tea with no added ingredients or black coffee.
- Dinner – Half portion of the drunken five-spice beef recipe, and 4 keto Snickerdoodle cookies for snack/dessert

Day 23 – the following meals will yield a total of 134 grams of fats, 80.4 grams of protein, 1543 calories, and 14.7 grams net carbs.

- Breakfast and lunch – Plenty of water. You can also drink tea with no added ingredients or black coffee.
- Dinner – Half portion of the Thai style peanut chicken recipe, 2 cups of spinach salad, and 3 almond lemon sandwich cakes for snack/dessert

Day 24 – the following meals will yield a total of 145.1 grams of fats, 72.6 grams of protein, 1600 calories, and 13.7 grams net carbs.

- Breakfast and lunch – Plenty of water. You can also drink tea with no added ingredients or black coffee.
- Dinner – Half portion of the cheesy creamed spinach recipe, 5 meatballs and chai spice mug cake with additional 2 tablespoons of heavy cream for snack/dessert

Day 25 – the following meals will yield a total of 145.1 grams of fats, 72.6 grams of protein, 1600 calories, and 13.7 grams net carbs.

- Breakfast and lunch – Plenty of water. You can also drink tea with no added ingredients or black coffee.
- Dinner – Half portion of the cheesy creamed spinach recipe, 5 meatballs and chai spice mug cake with additional 2 tablespoons of heavy cream for snack/dessert

Day 26 – the following meals will yield a total of 136.2 grams of fats, 77.9 grams of protein, 1517 calories, and 15.9 grams net carbs.

- Breakfast and lunch – Plenty of water. You can also drink tea with no added ingredients or black coffee.
- Dinner – A portion of roasted pecan green beans, 1/3 portion of the keto style Szechuan chicken recipe, and 4 almond lemon sandwich cakes with additional tablespoon of butter for snack/dessert

Day 27 – the following meals will yield a total of 136.2 grams of fats, 71.4 grams of protein, 1609 calories, and 14.8 grams net carbs.

- Breakfast and lunch – Plenty of water. You can also drink tea with no added ingredients or black coffee.
- Dinner – 1/3 portion of the vegetable medley recipe, 3 curry-rubbed chicken thighs, and 3 almond lemon sandwich cakes for snack/dessert

Day 28 – the following meals will yield a total of 133.3 grams of fats, 77.3 grams of protein, 1605 calories, and 10.3 grams net carbs.

- Breakfast and lunch – Plenty of water. You can also drink tea with no added ingredients or black coffee.
- Dinner – 2 cups of spinach salad, 1/4 portion of the wine and coffee beef stew recipe, 3 curry-rubbed chicken thighs, and chai spice mug cake with additional 3 tablespoons of heavy cream for snack/dessert

Day 29 – the following meals will yield a total of 132.9 grams of fats, 75.6 grams of protein, 1589 calories, and 19.7 grams net carbs.

- Breakfast and lunch – Plenty of water. You can also drink tea with no added ingredients or black coffee.
- Dinner – 1/2 portion of red pepper spinach salad, lemon and rosemary roasted chicken thighs, and 6 keto Snickerdoodle cookies for snack/dessert

Day 30

This is the beginning of week 5. You are done with fasting and you are already free to choose what to eat depending on your preferences and the leftovers that you still have in the fridge. If you want to continue fasting and found this to be beneficial, you can do so, but make sure that you take in the required daily macros.

Chapter 7 – 50 Ketogenic Fat-Burning Recipes

Here are the recipes that you can include in your daily meal plan, even now that you are on your own.

Keto Bombs Recipes for Snacks/Dessert

Keto bombs or fat bombs are ideal for dieters who need a boost of energy. They are also served to provide additional healthy fats and as snacks before or after every workout session.

#1: Simple Fat Bomb

The following ingredients will yield 24 pieces: For the coating, you will need 4 ounces of edible cocoa butter, a teaspoon of lemon extract, 2/3 cup of Swerve confectioners, and 1/4 teaspoon of sea salt. For the filling, you will need a cup of sweetener, 4 eggs, half a cup of lemon juice, 8 tablespoons of coconut oil, and a tablespoon of finely-grated lemon peel.

Melt the cocoa butter, add the sweetener, salt and extracts, and mix well. Pour this into your mold and place in the fridge for at least an hour. Prepare the lemon curd filling by whisking all the ingredients in a saucepan over medium heat. Continue whisking for 12 minutes, but do not allow it to boil. Strain it and transfer to a bowl. Put the bowl in another bowl that is filled with ice. Whisk occasionally and allow to cool completely. Make your truffles by putting a filling to each piece. Put them back to the fridge and allow to set before serving.

Nutritional Info: Each serving contains 10.1 grams of fat, 0.2 net carbs, 95 calories, and 1.1 grams of protein

#2 Lemon Fat Bombs

To make 16 servings of this delicious snack, you will need 1/4 cup extra virgin coconut oil (softened), 7.1 ounces of coconut butter (softened), up to 20 drops of sweetener, 2 teaspoons of lemon extract, and a pinch of salt.

Put all the ingredients in a bowl and mix until well-combined. Divide this into your molds and put in the fridge for an hour. This is ready to serve once set.

Nutritional Info: Each serving contains 11.9 grams of fat, 0.8 net carbs, 112 calories, and 0.76 gram of protein

#3 Basic Vanilla Fat Bombs

To make 16 servings, you'll need ¼ cup extra virgin coconut oil (softened), more or less 20 drops of sweetener, a pinch of salt, 7.1 ounces of coconut butter (softened), and a teaspoon of vanilla.

Basically, you will just have to follow the instructions for the previous recipe – combine everything in a sufficiently-sized container and then, divide the resulting mixture into your preferred molds. Put it in the fridge for about an hour and once set, it's good to eat.

Nutritional Info: Each serving contains 11.9 grams of fat, 0.8 net carbs, 112 calories, and 0.76 gram of protein

#4 Rose Water Fat Bombs

Here's a similar yet refreshingly unique variation of the basic fat bomb recipe. Instead of using lemon or vanilla, you'll be adding 2 teaspoons of rose water – giving your snack that Middle Eastern twist. Of course, you will still need ¼ cup extra virgin coconut oil (softened), more or less 20 drops of sweetener, a pinch of salt, and 7.1 ounces of coconut butter (softened) for a yield of 16 servings.

To prepare this mouth-watering keto treat, simply mix all the ingredients together and shape using a mold. Put them in the fridge for about an hour. Once everything has set, they're ready to tickle your taste buds.

Nutritional Info: Each serving contains 11.9 grams of fat, 0.8 net carbs, 112 calories, and 0.76 gram of protein

#5 Peppermint Fat Bombs

If you're craving for something that cools the tongue, try these peppermint fat bombs. To make 16 servings, you will need 1/4 cup extra virgin coconut oil (softened), 7.1 ounces of coconut butter (softened), up to 20 drops of sweetener, and a pinch of salt. You'll also need ½ teaspoon of peppermint extract.

Once you have gathered the ingredients, just combine everything in a bowl. Transfer the mixture into your preferred molds. When you're done, neatly place them in the fridge. They'll be ready to eat in approximately an hour.

Nutritional Info: Each serving contains 11.9 grams of fat, 0.8 net carbs, 112 calories, and 0.76 gram of protein

#6 Coco Cocoa Treat with Walnut

The following ingredients will yield 2 servings: 2 tablespoons of melted coconut oil, a tablespoon of sweetener, a tablespoon of unsweetened cocoa powder, a tablespoon of walnut halves (chopped and toasted), a tablespoon of heavy whipping cream, and a dash of sea salt.

Mix all ingredients in a bowl until you have a creamy sauce texture. Pour this on a sheet of wax paper and refrigerate until set. Break it into pieces and enjoy.

Nutritional Info: Each serving contains 17.77 grams of fat, 0.5 net carbs, 176.32 calories, and 1.26 grams of protein

#7 Coco Cocoa Treat with Brazil Nuts

To prepare 2 servings, you will need a pinch of sea salt, 2 tablespoons of melted coconut oil, a tablespoon of unsweetened cocoa powder, a tablespoon of Brazil nuts (chopped), a tablespoon of sweetener, and a tablespoon of heavy whipping cream.

Combine everything in a bowl. Don't stop mixing until the consistency becomes creamy. Transfer the mixture onto a sheet of wax paper. Refrigerate until set. Break apart and serve.

Nutritional Info: Each serving contains 18.02 grams of fat, 0.25 net carbs, 176.57 calories, and 1.26 grams of protein

#8 Coco Cocoa Treat with Pumpkin Seeds

Here's another variant of the coco cocoa treat recipe. To make 2 servings, you'll need 2 tablespoons of melted coconut oil, a tablespoon of sweetener, a tablespoon of unsweetened cocoa powder, a tablespoon of pumpkin seeds (roasted and chopped), a tablespoon of heavy whipping cream, and a dash of sea salt.

Put everything in a bowl and mix until creamy. Transfer the mixture onto a sheet of wax paper. Refrigerate and once set, break it into pieces.

Nutritional Info: Each serving contains 16.77 grams of fat, 0.25 net carbs, 169.82 calories, and 2.26 grams of protein

#9 Coco Cocoa Treat with Pecans

Pecans are among the top keto nuts, so you shouldn't be surprised to see them here. For a yield of 2 servings, you need to prepare a pinch of sea salt, a tablespoon of heavy whipping cream, a tablespoon of unsweetened cocoa powder, a tablespoon of Pecans (chopped), a tablespoon of sweetener, and 2 tablespoons of melted coconut oil.

Just like in the previous recipe, all you need to do is combine the ingredients until creamy, then put them on a sheet of wax paper before placing in the fridge. Once the mixture has set, break it into pieces and you're done.

Nutritional Info: Each serving contains 18.27 grams of fat, 0.25 net carbs, 177.57 calories, and 1.01 grams of protein

#10 Coco Cocoa Treat with Hazelnuts

The following ingredients will yield 2 servings: 2 tablespoons of melted coconut oil, a tablespoon of sweetener, a tablespoon of unsweetened cocoa powder, a tablespoon of hazelnuts (raw, chopped), a tablespoon of heavy whipping cream, and a dash of sea salt.

Place all the ingredients in a bowl. Combine until you come up with a creamy mixture. Get a sheet of wax paper and pour the mixture onto it. Put it in the fridge and wait until it hardens. When it has finally set, break it apart. Enjoy!

Nutritional Info: Each serving contains 17.52 grams of fat, 0.5 net carbs, 174.07 calories, and 1.26 grams of protein

#11 Coco Cocoa Treat with Flax Seeds

If you're really trying to push back your net carbs, this one's the ideal pick. To make 2 servings, you'll need 2 tablespoons of melted coconut oil, a tablespoon of unsweetened cocoa powder, a tablespoon of sweetener, a tablespoon of heavy whipping cream, a dash of sea salt, and a tablespoon of flax seeds (roasted).

Simply combine all ingredients until a creamy mixture is formed. Transfer it onto a sheet of wax paper and refrigerate for a while. When it has set, just break it apart. It's now ready to serve.

Nutritional Info: Each serving contains 15.77 grams of fat, 0 net carbs, 162.08 calories, and 2.01 grams of protein

#12 Special Vanilla Fat Bombs

These ingredients will yield 14 servings: 1/4 cup of softened butter, 1/4 cup of extra virgin coconut oil (melted), a cup of unsalted macadamia nuts, 2 teaspoons of sugar-free vanilla extract, 2 tablespoons of powdered sweetener, and up to 15 drops of Stevia extract.

Pulse the macadamia nuts in a blender until the consistency is smooth. Mix it with coconut oil and butter. Add the sweeteners and extracts and mix well. Pour into molds and put in the fridge for an hour to set.

Nutritional Info: Each serving contains 14.44 grams of fat, 0.6 net carbs, 132 calories, and 0.79 grams of protein

#13 Extra Special Vanilla Fat Bombs

To prepare 14 servings of this luxurious vanilla keto treat, you'll need 1/4 cup of softened butter, a cup of unsalted macadamia nuts, 2 tablespoons of powdered sweetener, up to 15 drops of Stevia extract, 1/4 cup of extra virgin coconut oil (melted), and 2 vanilla beans.

Put the macadamia in a blender and pulse until smooth. Add in both the butter and coconut oil. Pour in the sweeteners. Add the vanilla beans (you'll have to scrape them). Pulse again until a relatively even consistency is reached. Pour the mixture into your preferred molds. Refrigerate for an hour to set.

Nutritional Info: Each serving contains 14.44 grams of fat, 0.6 net carbs, 132 calories, and 0.79 grams of protein

#14 Sicilian Fat Bombs

This is perfect if you're looking for something a bit more interesting, given the Sicilian roots of its key flavor enhancer. To make 14 servings, you will need 1/4 cup of softened butter, 1/4 cup of extra virgin coconut oil (melted), a teaspoon of Fiori di Sicilia, 2 tablespoons of powdered sweetener, up to 15 drops of Stevia extract, and a cup of unsalted macadamia nuts.

Simply put everything in a food processor and pulse until well combined. Transfer the mixture into molds, then refrigerate. An hour should be enough for it to set.

Nutritional Info: Each serving contains 14.44 grams of fat, 0.6 net carbs, 132 calories, and 0.79 grams of protein

#15 Fat Bombs with Maple Syrup

If you're tired of using vanilla to flavor your fat bombs, you could try maple syrup – particularly the calorie-free kind. To prepare 14 servings, you'll need the following: 1/4 cup of softened butter, 1/4 cup of extra virgin coconut oil (melted), a cup of unsalted macadamia nuts, 2 teaspoons of no-calorie maple syrup, 2 tablespoons of powdered sweetener, and up to 15 drops of Stevia extract.

Just pulse the nuts in a blender, and then toss in the other ingredients. Pulse to combine. Put the resulting mixture into the molds you have prepared. Refrigerate then serve after an hour.

Nutritional Info: Each serving contains 14.44 grams of fat, 0.6 net carbs, 132 calories, and 0.79 grams of protein

#16 Pine Nuts and Vanilla Fat Bombs

These ingredients will yield 14 servings: 1/4 cup of softened butter, 1/4 cup of extra virgin coconut oil (melted), a cup of dry-roasted pine nuts (unsalted), 2 teaspoons of sugar-free vanilla extract, 2 tablespoons of powdered sweetener, and up to 15 drops of Stevia extract.

Pulse the pine nuts in a blender several times. Afterwards, combine it with coconut oil and butter. Put in the sweeteners and extracts and mix well. Pour into molds and place in the fridge. It should be ready to eat in an hour.

Nutritional Info: Each serving contains 13.73 grams of fat, 1.02 net carbs, 128.2 calories, and 1.28 grams of protein

#17 Vanilla and Pistachio Fat Bombs

To make 14 servings of this energy booster, you'll need to prepare 1/4 cup of softened butter, up to 15 drops of Stevia extract, 1/4 cup of extra virgin coconut oil (melted), 2 teaspoons of sugar-free vanilla extract, 2 tablespoons of powdered sweetener, and a cup of raw pistachio (unsalted, chopped).

Put the pistachio in a blender and pulse a few times. Add all the other ingredients and pulse again. Pour the mixture into molds then refrigerate. Your snack should be ready to eat in an hour.

Nutritional Info: Each serving contains 11.16 grams of fat, 1.5 net carbs, 112.63 calories, and 1.78 grams of protein

#18 Vanilla and Chia Fat Bombs

For 14 servings of this relatively light fat bomb recipe, simply prepare 1/4 cup of softened butter, 1/4 cup of extra virgin coconut oil (melted), 2 teaspoons of sugar-free vanilla extract, 2 tablespoons of powdered sweetener, 200 grams of chia seeds (lightly toasted), and up to 15 drops of Stevia extract.

Get your blender ready and put in all the ingredients except the chia seeds. Pulse a few times until the consistency becomes somewhat even. Pour in the chia seeds and mix. Transfer the mixture into your preferred molds. Refrigerate for approximately an hour.

Nutritional Info: Each serving contains 11.58 grams of fat, 1.24 net carbs, 132.7 calories, and 2.42 grams of protein

#19 Sacha Inchi Fat Bombs

Have a taste of Sacha Inchi by preparing this special fat bomb. To make 14 servings, you will need 1/4 cup of softened butter, 1/4 cup of extra virgin coconut oil (melted), 200 grams Sacha Inchi (crushed, dry roasted), 2 teaspoons of no-calorie maple syrup, 2 tablespoons of powdered sweetener, and up to 15 drops of Stevia extract.

Combine every ingredient in a food processor (except the Sacha Inchi) until consistency becomes even. Add in the nuts and mix. Place the mixture on appropriately-sized molds and refrigerate. Wait until set then serve.

Nutritional Info: Each serving contains 15.16 grams of fat, 0 net carbs, 160.42 calories, and 5.14 grams of protein

#20 Double Maple Fat Bombs

To prepare 14 servings of this sweet yet guilt-free dessert, you'll need 1/4 cup of softened butter, 1/4 cup of extra virgin coconut oil (melted), a cup of walnuts (pieces or chips), 4 teaspoons of zero-calorie maple syrup, 2 tablespoons of powdered sweetener, and up to 15 drops of Stevia extract.

Simply combine everything in a blender by pulsing several times. When done, transfer the mixture into molds. Place it in the fridge and it'll be ready in more or less an hour (check whether it has set).

Nutritional Info: Each serving contains 12.73 grams of fat, 0.57 net carbs, 119.35 calories, and 1.28 grams of protein

#21 Maple and Almond Fat Bombs

These ingredients will yield 14 servings: 2 tablespoons of powdered sweetener, up to 15 drops of Stevia extract, 1/4 cup of softened butter, 1/4 cup of extra virgin coconut oil (melted), a cup of almonds (slivered), and 2 teaspoons of calorie-free maple syrup.

Combine the coconut oil and butter, then add in the sweeteners and extracts. Once everything's well mixed, toss in the almonds. Distribute the mixture into your molds then place in the fridge. Your fat bombs should be ready in an hour.

Nutritional Info: Each serving contains 10.94 grams of fat, 0.81 net carbs, 107.7 calories, and 1.64 grams of protein

#22 Maple-Sesame Fat Bombs

To make 14 servings of this snack, you'll need 2 tablespoons of powdered sweetener, 1/4 cup of softened butter, up to 15 drops of Stevia extract, 1/4 cup of extra virgin coconut oil (melted), 2 teaspoons of calorie-free maple syrup, and a cup of sesame seeds.

Preparing this is easy. Just mix together all the ingredients, including the sesame seeds. Pour the mixture into molds. Put it in the fridge. It will be ready in about an hour.

Nutritional Info: Each serving contains 12.3 grams of fat, 1.31 net carbs, 122.2 calories, and 1.85 grams of protein

#23 Ginger Fat Bombs

To make 10 pieces of this treat, you will need 75 grams of softened coconut oil, 75 grams of softened coconut butter, 25 grams of unsweetened shredded coconut, half a teaspoon of dried powdered ginger, and a teaspoon of sweetener.

Combine all the ingredients and mix well. Make sure that the sweetener is dissolved and evenly distributed. Transfer the mixture into molds and refrigerate for at least 10 minutes.

Nutritional Info: Each serving contains 12.8 grams of fat, 2.2 grams of carbs, 120 calories, and 0.5 gram of protein

#24 Sugar-Free Dark Chocolate Keto Bombs

The following ingredients will yield 2 dozens: For the chocolate coating, you will need 2 ounces of unsweetened baking chocolate, a tablespoon of Swerve confectioner's powder, half an ounce of cocoa butter, 1/4 teaspoon of sugar-free vanilla extract, and 1/8 teaspoon of artificial sweetener. For the ganache filling, you will need 2 tablespoons plus 2 teaspoons of heavy cream, 5 ounces of low-carb chocolate, 1 1/4 teaspoons of chocolate extract, and half a teaspoon of chocolate extract.

Prepare the ganache first by melting the chocolate in a double boiler. Combine the vanilla and cream in a bowl and microwave for a couple of minutes. Combine the two mixtures and allow to temper for 5 minutes. Pour it in a bowl and cover with a plastic wrap. Chill it for several hours, or overnight. Once hard, it will be easier to manage. Form it into balls. Put the balls in a tray lined with parchment paper and refrigerate while you prepare the coating. For the chocolate coating, melt the cocoa butter and chocolate in a double boiler and then stir in the vanilla and sweeteners. Dip the balls in the melted topping. Allow to set and enjoy.

Nutritional Info: Each serving of 3 truffles contains 31 grams of fat, 13.8 grams of carbs, 1.3 grams net carbs, 292 calories, and 2.2 grams of protein

#25 Cinnamon and Coconut Fat Bombs

These ingredients can make 10 to 12 pieces of this treat: a cup of full-fat coconut milk, a cup of coconut butter, a teaspoon of vanilla extract, a teaspoon of artificial sweetener, half a teaspoon each of cinnamon and nutmeg, and a cup of shredded coconut.

Combine everything (except the shredded coconut) in a bowl, and put it in a double boiler. Stir the ingredients until melted and well-combined. Remove from heat and allow to cool a bit before putting it in the fridge to set. Form balls from the mixture and roll them in the shredded coconut. Arrange the balls on a tray and refrigerate before serving.

Nutritional Info: The whole recipe contains 341 calories, 31.9 grams of fat, 12.8 grams of carbs, 5.3 grams net carbs, 292 calories, and 3.3 grams of protein

#26 Not Your Caveman's Chili

Cut a pound of stew meat into small cubes and process another pound of the meat in the food processor into ground beef. Sauté both and continue cooking in a slow cooker.

Sauté chopped onion, green pepper, and a tablespoon of minced garlic. In a bowl, combine 2 tablespoons each of olive oil, soy sauce and chili powder, as well as 2 teaspoons each of paprika and fish sauce. Also add a teaspoon each of Worcestershire and oregano, half a teaspoon of cayenne pepper, 1 1/2 teaspoons of cumin, and 1/3 cup of tomato paste. Put the mixture into the slow cooker, along with a cup of beef broth. Mix and allow to simmer for 2 hours and 30 minutes on high. Remove the cover and continue to simmer for another 30 minutes.

Nutritional Info: The recipe makes 4 servings. Each serving contains 17.8 grams of fats, 398 calories, 51.8 grams of protein, and 5.3 grams net carbs

#27 Flaming Cayenne Chili

To prepare this, you'll need a pound of each of cubed and ground stew meat. Sauté those for a bit then transfer to a slow cooker.

Now, sauté some green pepper and chopped onion, as well as a tablespoon of minced garlic. Mix 2 tablespoons each of soy sauce, chili powder, and olive oil. Add 2 teaspoons each of fish sauce and paprika, as well as a 2 teaspoons of Cayenne pepper. Mix again. Put a teaspoon each Worcestershire and oregano, 1 1/2 teaspoons of cumin, and 1/3 cup of tomato paste.

Once you've mixed the ingredients, put them in the slow cooker. Add a cup of beef broth. Give it a stir and let simmer for 2 hours and 30 minutes on high. Remove the lid and simmer for half an hour more.

Nutritional Info: The recipe makes 4 servings. Each serving contains 17.8 grams of fats, 398 calories, 51.8 grams of protein, and 5.3 grams net carbs

#28 Tongue-Friendly Chili

If you're not that into spicy food, this chili recipe should be perfect for you. To make it, start by sautéing a pound each of cubed and ground stew meat. After a few minutes, put them in a slow cooker.

Once you're done with those steps, combine the following ingredients in a bowl: 2 tablespoons each of soy sauce and olive oil, a tablespoon of chili powder, 2 teaspoons each of paprika and fish sauce, a teaspoon each of oregano and Worcestershire sauce, and 1/3 cup of tomato paste.

Sauté a tablespoon of minced garlic combined with some green pepper slices and chopped onion. Add these to the mixture and put everything in the slow cooker. Pour in a cup of beef broth, stir, then close the lid. Simmer for 2 hours and 30 minutes on high. Open the lid then simmer for half an hour, and it's done.

Nutritional Info: The recipe makes 4 servings. Each serving contains 17.8 grams of fats, 398 calories, 51.8 grams of protein, and 5.3 grams net carbs

#29 Bulletproof Coffee

There are two ways to take this – drink it like regular coffee or drink the coffee and eat the other ingredients. To make the beverage, brew a cup of coffee. Drop a tablespoon of butter in the coffee, along with a tablespoon of coconut oil. Mix and then add a tablespoon of heavy cream. Mix everything using a hand blender until well-combined.

Nutritional Info: One serving contains 30 grams of fats, 1 gram net carbs, and 273 calories

#30 Sweet-Spiced Coffee

If you're getting tired of the typical bulletproof blend, you should try this recipe. Simply brew a cup of coffee, then add in a tablespoon of butter. Put a tablespoon of coconut oil as well. Give it a stir while adding a tablespoon of heavy cream. Now, add 2-4 drops of liquid stevia. Use a hand blender to properly combine everything. Transfer into a cup and add a pinch or two of cardamom.

Nutritional Info: One serving contains 30 grams of fats, 1 gram net carbs, and 273 calories

#31 Bulletproof Coffee with Cinnamon

Prepare a cup of coffee and add a tablespoon each of butter and coconut oil in it. Drop a tablespoon of heavy cream and use a hand blender to mix thoroughly. Get 1/8 teaspoon of cinnamon and carefully sprinkle it on top.

Nutritional Info: One serving contains 30 grams of fats, 1 gram net carbs, and 273 calories

#32 Apple Pie Morning Brew

Brew a cup of coffee and once again, add a tablespoon each of coconut oil and butter, as well as heavy cream. Add a dash of cinnamon, a pinch of nutmeg, ginger, and cardamom, and a tiny sprinkle of allspice. Put in 2 drops of liquid stevia. Combine with a hand blender and enjoy.

Nutritional Info: One serving contains 30 grams of fats, 1 gram net carbs, and 273 calories

#33 Bulletproof Coffee with Turmeric

They say turmeric comes with lots of health benefits, so why not add it to your coffee? Simply brew a cup and add the other necessary ingredients (a tablespoon each of butter, coconut oil, and heavy cream). Now, put in 1/8 teaspoon of turmeric powder. Mix with a handle blender.

Nutritional Info: One serving contains 30 grams of fats, 1 gram net carbs, and 273 calories

#34 Pepper-Powered Bulletproof Coffee

Get 1/8 teaspoon of black pepper and mix it with your ground coffee beans. Brew as usual and once done, add in a tablespoon each of coconut oil, butter, and heavy cream. Use a hand blender to evenly combine.

Nutritional Info: One serving contains 30 grams of fats, 1 gram net carbs, and 273 calories

#35 Simple Lunch Salad

This can be done by combining all the wet ingredients in a bowl and combining 2 cups of spinach and 100 grams of beef (cooked, shredded) in another bowl. Only mix the two when you are ready to eat. The wet ingredients that you will need to prepare the dressing are 1 1/2 teaspoons of mustard, 4 tablespoons of olive oil, and zest of 1/4 lemon.

Nutritional Info: One serving contains 61 grams of fats, 3.3 grams net carbs, 30 grams protein, and 667 calories

#36 Cheesy Chicken Lunch Salad

To prepare this salad, you'll need 100 grams of chicken meat (diced, cooked) and 2 cups of spinach. Simply toss those ingredients together and place them in a bowl. Now, combine 4 tablespoons of olive oil, 1 1/2 teaspoons of mustard, and zest of 1/4 lemon. Drizzle the mixture on top of the chicken and greens. Sprinkle a tablespoon of parmesan on top, and you're done.

Nutritional Info: One serving contains 69.4 grams of fats, 2 grams net carbs, 29.9 grams protein, and 753 calories

#37 Lunch Salad with Lamb

To make this dish, you will need 2 cups of spinach and 100 grams of lamb meat (ground, cooked). Mix them together and place in a bowl. Afterwards, mix 1 1/2 teaspoons of mustard, 4 tablespoons olive oil, and zest of 1/4 lemon, then drizzle the mixture on the meat and greens. Toss and then add a pinch of ground black pepper before serving.

Nutritional Info: One serving contains 77 grams of fats, 2 grams net carbs, 18 grams protein, and 774 calories

#38 Crunchy Lunch Salad

You'll need the following to make a single serving of this salad: 2 cups of spinach, 5 slices of bacon (pan-fried, crisped, chopped), 1 1/2 teaspoons of mustard, 4 tablespoons of olive oil, and zest of 1/4 lemon.

Combine the last three ingredients to make the dressing. Place the spinach in a bowl and drizzle the dressing over it. Top with bacon.

Nutritional Info: One serving contains 70.5 grams of fats, 2.5 grams net carbs, 16 grams protein, and 707 calories

#39 Wild Lunch Salad

To prepare this, you will need 2 cups of spinach, 100 grams of venison (ground, pan-broiled), 4 tablespoons of olive oil, zest of 1/4 lemon, 1 1/2 teaspoons of mustard. Toss together the first two ingredients in a sufficiently-sized bowl. Create the dressing using the last three ingredients on the list. Drizzle over venison and spinach. Serve and enjoy.

Nutritional Info: One serving contains 62 grams of fats, 2 grams net carbs, 27 grams protein, and 679 calories

#40 Three-Cheese Lunch Salad

Combine all the wet ingredients in a bowl, as well as combine 2 cups of spinach and 100 grams of beef (cooked, shredded) in another bowl. Only mix the two right before serving. The wet ingredients that you will need for this recipe are 1 1/2 teaspoons of mustard, zest of 1/4 lemon, and 4 tablespoons of olive oil.

Once you've mixed the contents of the two bowls, top with a tablespoon each of Cheddar, Parmesan, and Parmigiano.

Nutritional Info: One serving contains 64.83 grams of fats, 3.3 grams net carbs, 34.82 grams protein, and 737 calories

#41 Tongue-Tickler Lunch Salad

You'll need these to make a single serving: 2 cups of spinach, 5 slices of bacon (pan-fried, crisped, chopped), 4 tablespoons of olive oil, zest of 1/4 lemon, and 1 1/2 teaspoons of mustard.

Mix together the last three ingredients to prepare the dressing. Transfer the spinach in a bowl and drizzle the dressing over it. Top with bacon and add a dash of Cayenne powder.

Nutritional Info: One serving contains 70.5 grams of fats, 2.5 grams net carbs, 16 grams protein, and 707 calories

#42 Buffalo Lunch Salad

Combine 4 tablespoons of olive oil, 1 1/2 teaspoons of mustard, and zest of 1/4 lemon in a bowl, and then set aside. Now, mix together 2 cups of spinach and 100 grams of buffalo meat (ground, cooked). Drizzle the dressing over the greens and meat, and it's ready to eat.

Nutritional Info: One serving contains 69.9 grams of fats, 2 grams net carbs, 19.7 grams protein, and 715 calories

#43 Lunch Salad with Fresh Mozzarella

To make a serving of this delectable salad, just combine 4 tablespoons of olive oil, zest of 1/4 lemon, and 1 1/2 teaspoons of mustard. Drizzle that over 2 cups of spinach. Add 100 grams of diced Mozzarella (low sodium) on top and serve.

Nutritional Info: One serving contains 71 grams of fats, 5.1 grams net carbs, 29 grams protein, and 772 calories

#44 Roasted Pecan Green Beans

Process 1/4 cup of pecans in a food processor until chopped. Put them in a bowl and mix with 2 tablespoons of Parmesan cheese, the zest of 1/2 lemon, a teaspoon of minced garlic, 2 tablespoons of olive oil, half a teaspoon of red pepper flakes, and half a pound of green beans.

Arrange them in a foiled baking sheet and bake in a preheated oven at 450 degrees Fahrenheit for 25 minutes. Allow to cool before serving.

Nutritional Info: The recipe will yield 3 servings, with each serving containing 16.8 grams of fats, 182 calories, 3.7 grams of protein, and 3.3 grams net carbs

#45 Roasted Almond Green Beans

Place 1/4 cup of slivered almonds in a bowl and toss together with the zest of 1/2 lemon, a teaspoon of minced garlic, 2 tablespoons of Parmesan cheese, 2 tablespoons of olive oil, half a pound of green beans, and half a teaspoon of red pepper flakes.

Put everything in a foiled baking sheet. Bake for 25 minutes at 450 degrees Fahrenheit. Let cool and serve.

Nutritional Info: The recipe will yield 3 servings, with each serving containing 14.71 grams of fats, 174 calories, 4.77 grams of protein, and 3.71 grams net carbs

#46 Green Beans with Macadamia

To prepare this dish, you'll have to first put the following ingredients in a bowl: a teaspoon of minced garlic, zest of 1/2 lemon, 2 tablespoons of Parmesan cheese, 2 tablespoons of olive oil, half a teaspoon of red pepper flakes, half a pound of green beans, and 1/4 cup of macadamia nuts. Give the ingredients a toss before placing them in a foiled baking sheet. Bake at 450 degrees Fahrenheit for 25 minutes. Allow to cool before serving.

Nutritional Info: The recipe will yield 3 servings, with each serving containing 18.8 grams of fats, 199.42 calories, 3.77 grams of protein, and 3.46 grams net carbs

#47 Green Beans with Chia Seeds

Toss together 2 tablespoons of Parmesan cheese, the zest of 1/2 lemon, a teaspoon of minced garlic, 2 tablespoons of olive oil, half a teaspoon of red pepper flakes, and half a pound of green beans.

Place them in a foiled baking sheet. Put in the oven for 25 minutes at 450 degrees Fahrenheit. Remove from the oven, top with an ounce of chia seeds (toasted), allow to cool, and serve.

Nutritional Info: The recipe will yield 3 servings, with each serving containing 16.3 grams of fats, 165.25 calories, 4.42 grams of protein, and 3.54 grams net carbs

#48 Green Beans with Brazil Nuts

Combine ¼ cup of Brazil nuts (chopped), half a pound of green beans, 2 tablespoons of Parmesan cheese, a teaspoon of minced garlic, 2 tablespoons of olive oil, half a teaspoon of red pepper flakes, and the zest of 1/2 lemon in a bowl.

Put the ingredients in a foiled baking sheet. Bake at 450 degrees Fahrenheit for 25 minutes. Transfer to another container and allow to cool.

Nutritional Info: The recipe will yield 3 servings, with each serving containing 17.63 grams of fats, 191.91 calories, 4.44 grams of protein, and 3.38 grams net carbs

#49 Toasted Flax Green Beans

To prepare this dish, simply mix together half a pound of green beans, a teaspoon of minced garlic, 2 tablespoons of olive oil, 2 tablespoons of Parmesan cheese, half a teaspoon of red pepper flakes, and the zest of 1/2 lemon in a bowl.

Put these in the oven and bake on a foiled baking sheet for 25 minutes at 450 degrees Fahrenheit. Once done, transfer to another container and top with 3 tablespoons of toasted flax seeds.

Nutritional Info: The recipe will yield 3 servings, with each serving containing 14.6 grams of fats, 174.25 calories, 4.76 grams of protein, and 3.08 grams net carbs

#50 Crispy Curry-Rubbed Chicken Thigh

The following ingredients will yield 1 serving. If you are following the menu plan on this book and you are already in the 4th week, make sure that you add an additional chicken thigh: 2 chicken thighs, a tablespoon of olive oil, half a teaspoon each of salt and yellow curry, 1/4 teaspoon each of garlic powder, cumin and paprika, 1/8 teaspoon each of coriander, chili powder, cayenne pepper and allspice, and a pinch each of cinnamon, cardamom and ginger.

Lay the chicken thighs on a baking sheet wrapped with foil and rub them with olive oil. Mix all the spices in a bowl and rub all sides of the chicken thighs with the mixture. Make sure that you coat all sides liberally. Bake the chicken in a preheated oven at 425 degrees Fahrenheit for an hour. Allow to cool before serving.

Nutritional Info: The recipe contains 39.8 grams of fats, 555 calories, 42.3 grams of protein, and 1.3 grams net carbs.

Conclusion

Thanks again for taking the time to download this book!

You should now have a good understanding of what the ketogenic diet is all about. Hopefully, you'll be able to successfully integrate it into your lifestyle.

If you enjoyed this book, please take the time to leave me a review on Amazon. I appreciate your honest feedback, and it really helps me to continue producing high quality books.

Simply CLICK HERE to leave a review, or check out my website www.fatadapteddoc.com.

Other Books By This Author

I hope you enjoyed reading this book! I have put allot of work into studying and researching Intermittent Fasting, Ketogenic Diets, Low Carb High Fat Lifestyles, Fat Adaptation, and Heart Rate Training.

I have some other books that I have written on Amazon that I think you might be interested in. Below is a list of my other books, along with direct links to their pages on Amazon.

Intermittent Fasting: 6 effective methods to lose weight, build muscle, increase your metabolism, get ketogenic, and get healthy

Ketogenic Diet Plan: 30 Day Meal Plan, 50 Ketogenic Fat Burning Recipes for Rapid Weight Loss and Unstoppable Energy

Low Carb High Fat 101: 20+ Best Recipes and Weekly LCHF Meal Plan, LCHF Explained, Ketogenic Diet and Fat Adapted Training

About the Author

Dr. Dan Foss graduated from Western States Chiropractic College in 2003. His fresh outlook on health, nutrition, and exercise has helped thousands of people not only get well but stay well for a lifetime. His goal as a Chiropractor is to help educate and empower people to understand how the human body works so that they can make the best decisions regarding their health and well-being. Over the last 13 years he has practiced Chiropractic and the last 7 years has owned and operated Pura Vida Chiropractic, a wellness center based in San Antonio, Texas. When not practicing he is a father, husband, coach, mentor, and amateur endurance athlete.

Thank You

Maybe you picked up multiple books on the topic of ketogenic diets and gave mine a shot. One of the greatest gifts one can give is the gift of knowledge and sharing this knowledge was my ultimate goal in creating this book. If you enjoyed it please share you review on Amazon so that other readers can enjoy it as well.

Your feedback allows me to continue to help and serve others and really help make a difference in our world. So if you enjoyed it, please let me know!

Made in the USA
San Bernardino, CA
28 August 2017